To all the survivors

for believing you can

and for Den, Mom and Dad, and Jewls K.,

for always believing in me

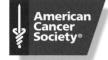

I Can Survive

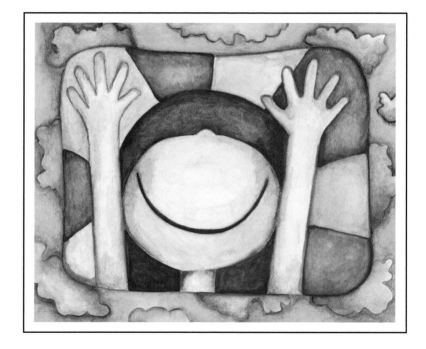

Written and illustrated by
Jennifer May Allen

For the Survivor in Each of Us!

I can survive, reaching arms high,

finding sunrise sky.

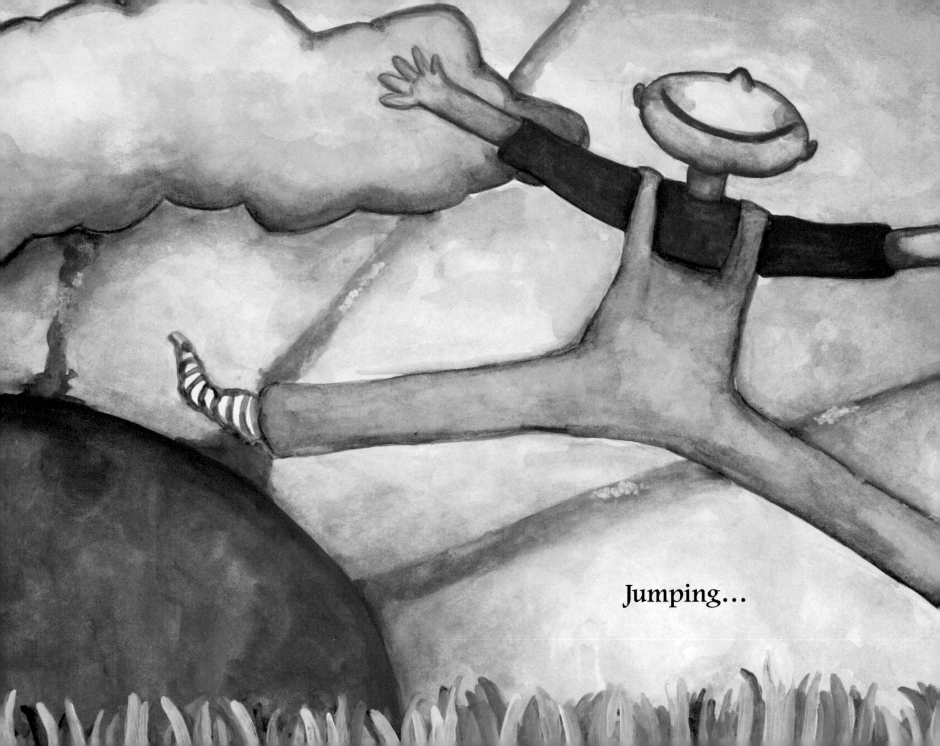

Jumping…

I cartwheel three times,
waving pompoms
when I don't even score.

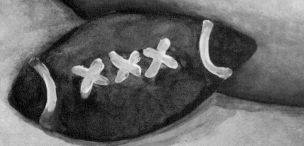

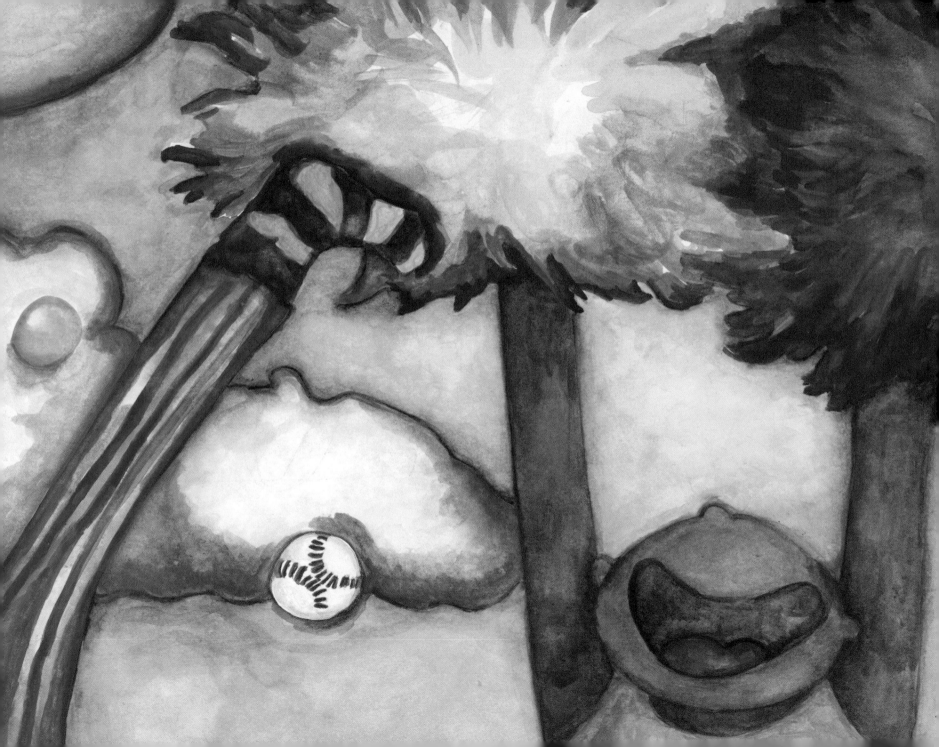

On boring Tuesdays
I wear tattered overalls,
a smile and hello.

Thursdays are for plucking
dandelions in parking lots and
baking Mama's chocolate cake.

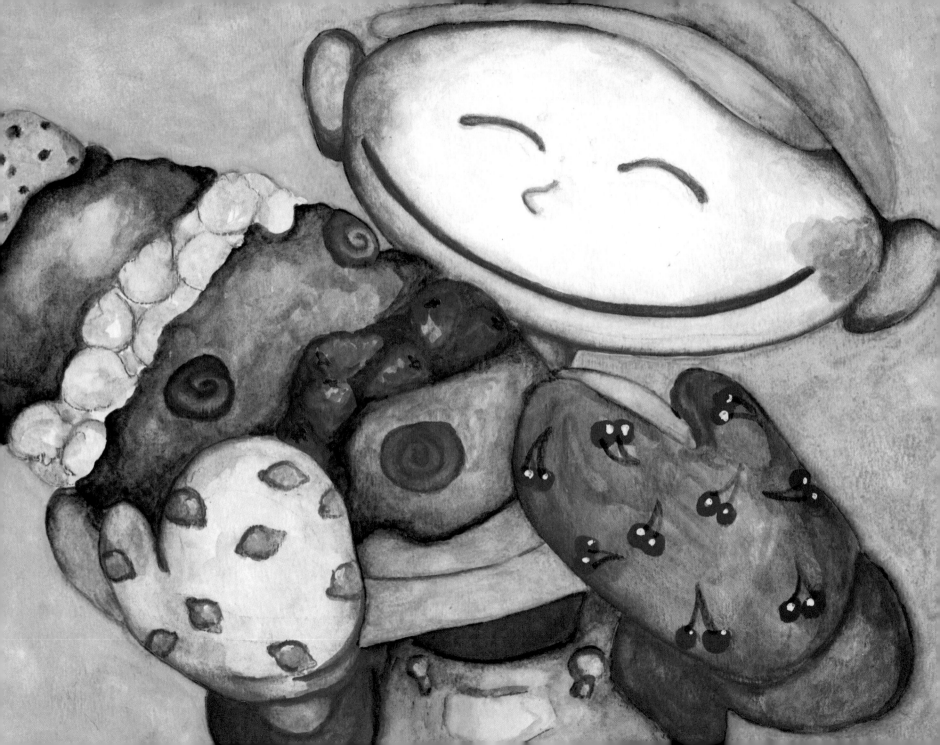

As early July fireworks boom above my humid sleeping bag, clumsily I will trace our hands in thick line.

I will hold you this way, we together in crayon.

I can open my heart
and feel your love,

pet my precocious cat
and walk my bouncing dog.

Don't bother me at two in the afternoon...

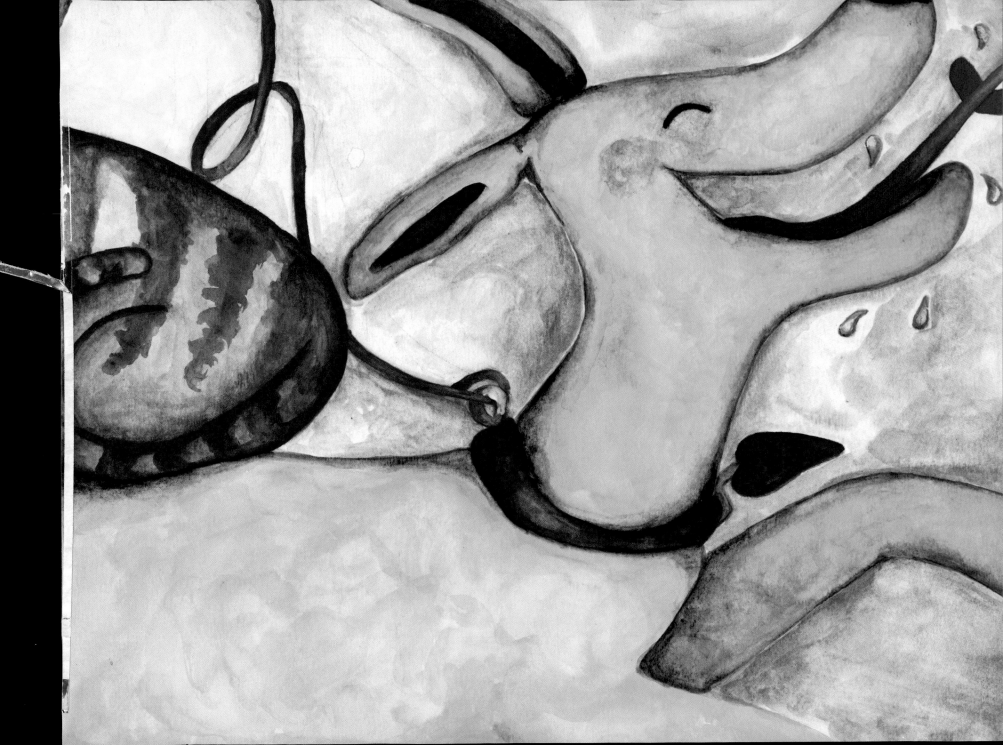

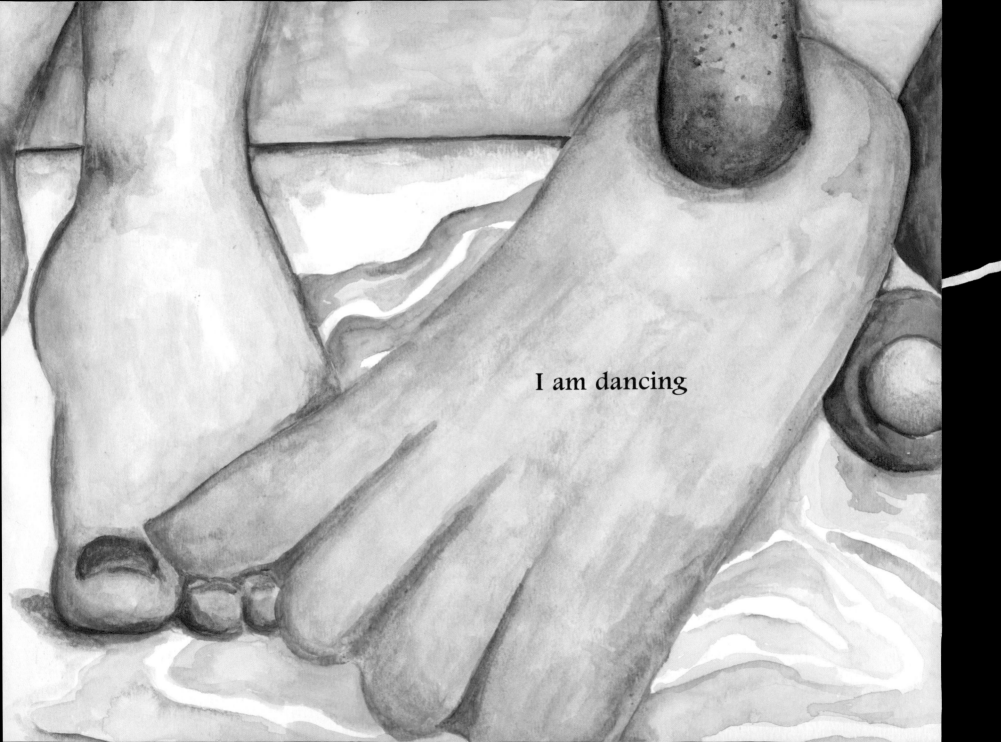

I am dancing

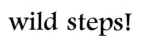

wild steps!

On Wednesday mornings I realize I may be lost

and drowse in dampening caves.

Circling everywhere

but home, I only find
that sometimes I
do need help.

Laughing, you smell like raspberry muffins, and suddenly alone disappears into your hugs.

I can survive!

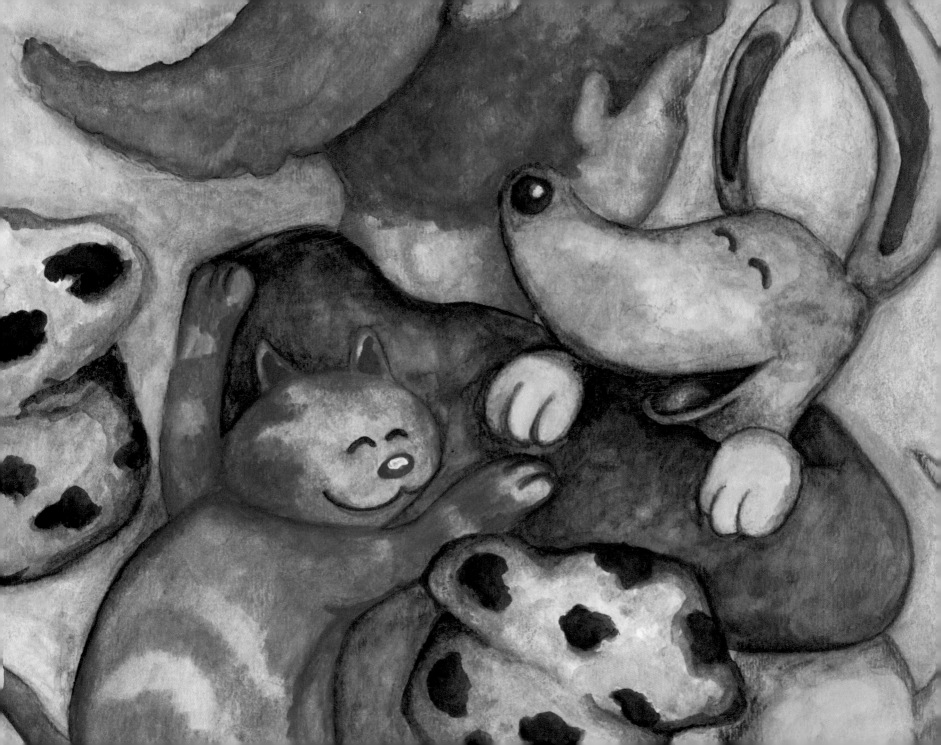

Inhaling giggles,
   nothing can stop that.
      Smiling,

I paint loud
everything.

I am always me.

I will always be me.

Even when I am scared,

running five miles away, parachuting

from airplanes and swimming

into the deepest swirls,

I remember…

I can survive!

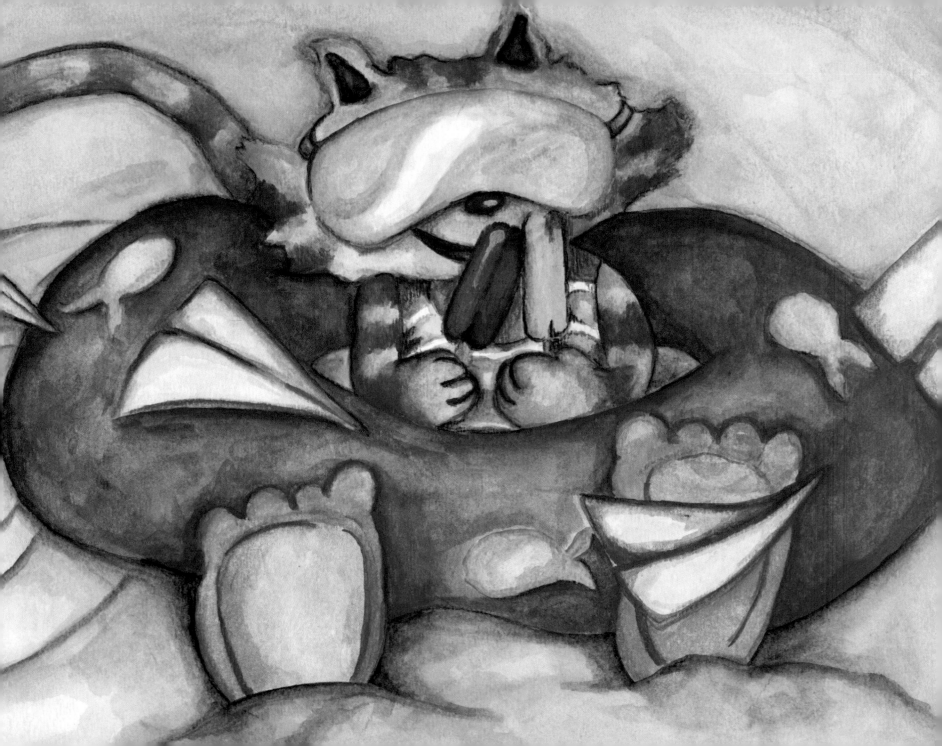

I am still here.

I am strong.

My heart is true.

I love me.

I love you, you, you,

and forever

you.

I will survive.

I will be me

no matter what or where.

I may change outside

and even in...

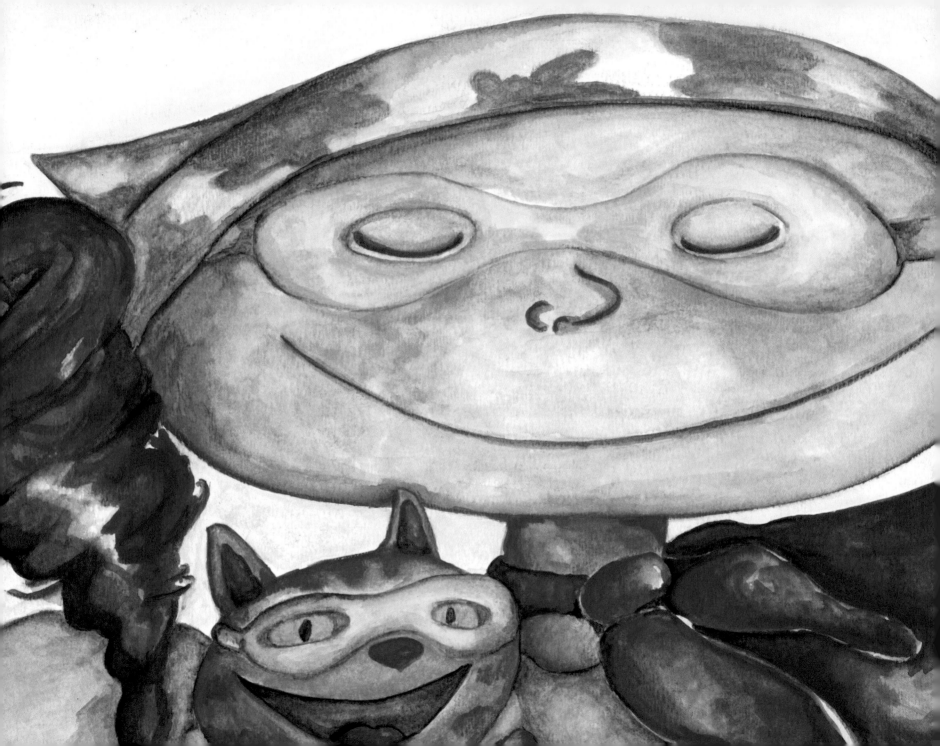

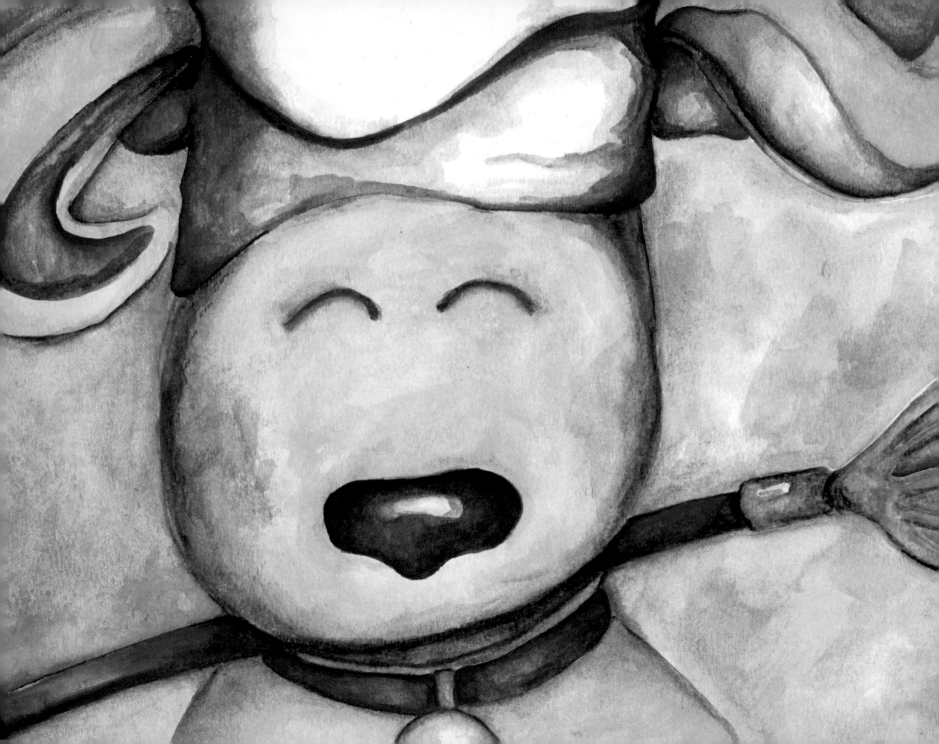

But I will always, each and every day,
love to lick the brownie spoon.
Nothing can change that.

I can survive.

I will survive.

Speaking,

    breathing,

        tasting,

            hearing,

                feeling,

                    believing,

I can survive.

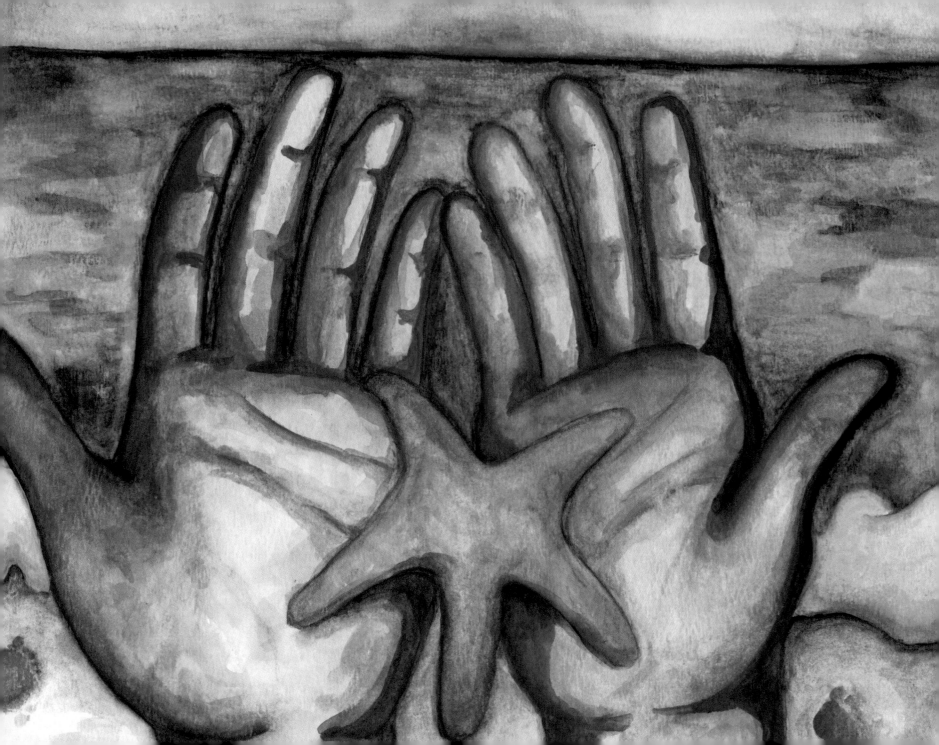

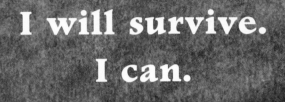

I will survive.
I can.

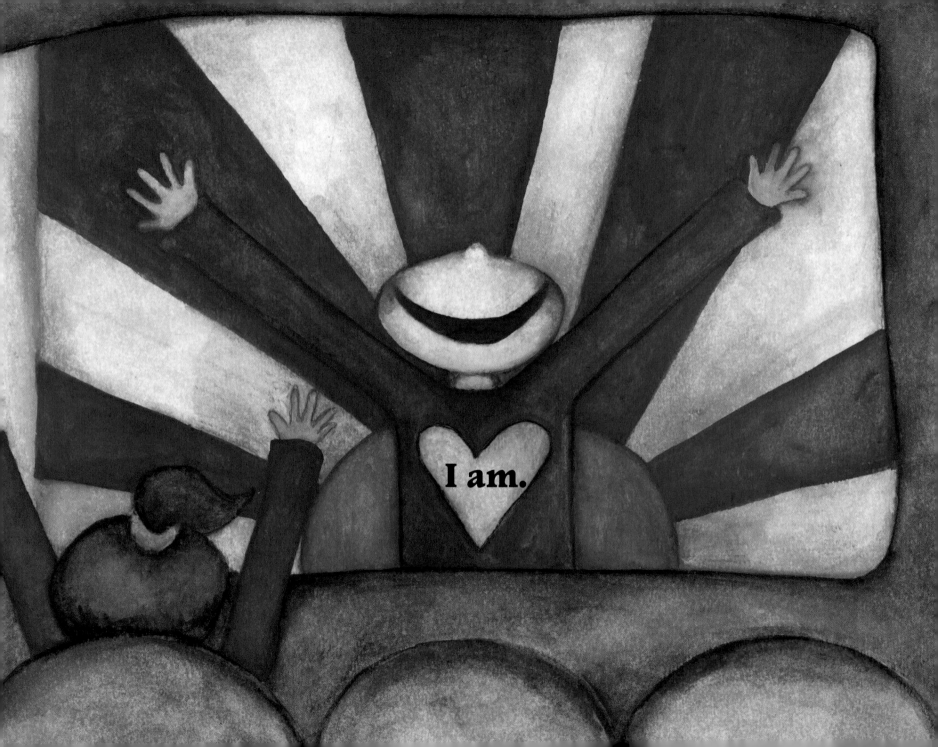

Published by the
American Cancer Society
Health Promotions
1599 Clifton Road NE
Atlanta, Georgia 30329 USA

Printed in Mexico
5 4 3 2 1   07 08 09 10 11

Library of Congress Cataloging-in-Publication Data

Allen, Jennifer M. (Jennifer May), 1980-
   I can survive : for the survivor in each of us! / written and illustrated by Jennifer May Allen.
      p. cm.
   ISBN-13: 978-0-944235-76-8
   ISBN-10: 0-944235-76-X
   1. Cancer—Popular works. I. Title.

RC254.5.A45 2007
362.196'9940092—dc22
                                    2006036302

MANAGING EDITOR
Rebecca Teaff

BOOK PUBLISHING MANAGER
Candace Magee

DIRECTOR, BOOK PUBLISHING
Len Boswell

STRATEGIC DIRECTOR, CONTENT
Chuck Westbrook

For more information about cancer, contact your American Cancer Society
at 1-800-ACS-2345 or www.cancer.org

For special sales, email us at
trade.sales@cancer.org